Table of Contents

What is an Endomorph?

The classification of different body types was introduced in the 1940s by American researcher and psychologist William Sheldon. Through his research he concluded that, based on our skeletal frame and body composition, we all have inherited body types that determine whether we're leaner, heavier, or somewhere in between. Because of this inherited body type, reaching weight loss and fitness goals often requires an individualized program.

Endomorphs are said to have a higher percentage of body fat with less muscle mass.

They're often heavier and rounder, but not necessarily obese. Because of their physical makeup, people with endomorphic bodies are more sensitive to calorie consumption than people with other body types. Endomorphs must carefully watch their food intake to ensure they don't consume more calories than they burn. Other characteristics include a larger frame and an inability to drop weight.

These characteristics differ from the other two body types: ectomorph and mesomorph. People with an ectomorph somatotype have higher metabolisms, which means they can eat more and gain little weight. They also have smaller joints, a smaller body size, and a narrower frame.

The mesomorph somatotype, on the other hand, is in between ectomorph and endomorph. These individuals may have a larger skeletal frame, but a lower percentage of body fat. They can typically gain muscle and lose weight easily.

Endomorph Diet Help You Lose Weight

Whether you're looking to drop excess pounds or add some muscle definition, getting results involves maintaining a healthy diet and regular exercise. But depending on your body type, some diet and workout plans may work better than others.

If you have a higher percentage of body fat and little muscle definition, you may have what is known as an endomorph body. Some people with endomorphic bodies struggle with weight loss. However, the key is understanding how your body type differs from other types and knowing what to eat and what not to eat.

What Endomorph Should Eat

If you have an endomorphic body and you're looking to lose weight or gain muscle definition, you may consider a fitness plan and diet that's specific to your body type.

According to the diet's theory, endomorphs have slower metabolisms. Since you don't burn calories as fast as ectomorphs and mesomorphs, excess calories are more likely to convert to fat. Some believe you're also less tolerable to carbohydrates, so the best diet for your body type may be one with a higher fat and protein intake and a lower carbohydrate intake, such as the paleo diet. This diet can help you lose body fat while keeping your energy level up.

Good Sources of Fats and Proteins

• Macadamia nuts

- Olive oil

- Beef

- Egg yolk

- Fatty fish

- Walnuts

- Cheese

You don't have to avoid carbohydrates. Carbs are an excellent source of energy. Removing carbs from your diet can trigger sluggishness and fatigue. If too extreme, a low-carb diet can also lead to gastrointestinal problems and ketosis. The trick is choosing the right kind of carbs. Focus on complex carbohydrates like vegetables, including starchy vegetables like potatoes and tubers, legumes, whole grains, and fruits.

Limit your intake of simple carbohydrates. These foods are high in sugar and calories, which can cause fat storage. Simple carbohydrates include white bread, white rice, pasta, cakes, and cookies.

Fruit is a healthy addition to any diet program. If you're carb-sensitive, eat fruit in moderation. According to the American Council of Exercise, you should follow this formula when planning your daily meals:

• 30 percent carbohydrates

- 35 percent protein

- 35 percent fat

Portion control is also important when reducing body fat as an endomorph. This helps you avoid excess calorie consumption. Eating 200 to 500 fewer calories than you normally consume will also help you reach your weight loss goal.

According to proponents of the diet — because endomorphs have a harder time losing body fat — dieting alone may not be enough to lose weight. Incorporate physical activity into your daily routine, which is a common recommendation for anyone looking to improve health.

An effective fitness plan includes a combination of weight training and cardio training.

What Research Say About Diet and Body Type

There's been little research to date that's studied how diet should be modified based on somatotype to achieve specific results.

Losing weight can seem like an uphill battle when your efforts don't pay off. Understanding your individual body type, as well as the unique challenges faced by endomorphs, may help you drop pounds and hit your fitness goals.

Maintain a low intake of refined carbs, get plenty of regular physical activity, and practice portion control. These are all healthy behaviors recommended for most people. Sticking with this routine may help you shed excess pounds — and keep the weight off.

Weight Loss Plan for an Endomorph Body Type

Endomorph body types tend to have a slower metabolism meaning that losing weight can be more of a challenge. When it comes to losing weight, it is best to choose a plan that suits your body type, as this ensures that the nutrition values are suited to the way your body works and is to your advantage. Rather than following a strict diet for so many days, it is best to choose a weight loss plan that will allow you to lose weight healthily over time and combine with a little exercise to keep your body fit and healthy, so here at OneHowTo, we're going to tell you the best weight loss plan for an endomorph body type.

Steps to Follow

No matter what your body type, it is important to remember when it comes to losing weight, a good balance of healthy eating and exercise will do your body much better than crash dieting. Starving your body of nutrients is not a good long term plan for keeping yourself in shape! Weight loss can be a slow process so patience is key!

Step One

To start with, decide on an exercise regime that will fit around your schedule that you are likely to stick to. Cardio is best for endomorph body types as it keeps you active and burns calories which is great if you are working towards weight loss. Organise yourself so you can go running in the morning or after work, or a gym session every other day. Organisation is important if you want to stick to your weight loss plan.

Step Two

Cardio training for an endomorph should be 30-60 minutes per session, two or three times per week. Start with less and build yourself up. Make sure cardio training is steady state, don't push yourself to reach goals that you aren't ready for, you'll get there soon enough!

Try to incorporate different types of cardio into your fitness routine. Endomorphs will benefit from a long term fitness plan so mix up your exercise so you don't get bored, alternate between running or cycling to keep things new. Work on a 30 minute high intensity interval workout for no less than 30 minutes, 3 times per week.

Step Three

Weight training can also aid weight loss and fuel the burning of fats. Work on larger muscles such as your legs, back and arms doing 15 reps per 2 sets. Again, start smaller and work your way up.

Step Four

When it comes to a diet plan, individuals with endomorph body types are best focusing their meals around proteins and fats rather than carbohydrates. Whilst it is important to still give your body good carbs coming from foods such as quinoa - try and work these into a meal after a work out. Stay away from breads and white rice and pasta. Take a look at the article how to organize a healthy diet for some ideas!

Step Five

Endomorph body types tend to mainly process the sugar in carbs, and by eating these whilst you're body is still pumped from the work out, they are more likely to be turned into energy rather than unhelpful sugar you want to avoid in weight loss.

Step Six

Eating a good amount of vegetables with each meal will also promote weight loss. It is sometimes harder for people with an endomorph body type to develop a lean look, so cutting out the 'bad' sugars from cookies and cakes will be beneficial. Eating fruits and vegetables mean energy will be released slower which will also prevent you feeling hungry and snacking. Eat fruit moderately as these foods still contain sugar but fruit is good to have to hand if you do feel yourself wanting a nibble throughout the day.

Step Seven

Keeping active is key when it comes to weight loss, no matter what your body type - but it is particularly important for endomorph. As summer is coming up, try taking a walk rather than watching TV, you will notice the changes in your body! It can also help to work out with a friend or partner if you tend to lack the motivation.

A Simple Way to Finally Lose Weight

Do you ever feel like you only have to look at food and your body naturally puts on weight that is super hard to drop?

If this sounds like you, read on, because this book is all about the endomorph diet plan.

Next time you find yourself in a group of people, look around. You'll hopefully notice that no two people are built quite the same.

But if you look long enough, you'll notice most people can be sorted into groups of similar body types.

Everyone knows the importance of a healthy diet and fitness plan, but did you know that depending on your body type, some women's diets may work better than others?

What are Somatotypes?

Somatotyping is a classification system that was developed in the 1940s by psychologist, William Herbert Sheldon, to categorize the human body into three loose groupings, or somatotypes.

Somatotypes in Three Categories

Ectomorphs

Usually have long, lean bodies and have a fast metabolism. They often have a hard time gaining weight and muscle.

Mesomorphs

Naturally muscular and have the ability to lose weight or gain weight easily. They're often described as having athletic builds.

Endomorphs

This group is usually characterized by a larger bone structure. They generally store up fat easily and often struggle with weight loss.

Sheldon's research indicated that because we all have different inherited body types, reaching our fitness and weight loss goals requires different approaches, depending on our somatotype.

Most people are a blend of two somatotypes, but will usually have one that is more dominant.

Endomorph Diet Plan

Since ectomorphs are usually naturally lean, and mesomorphs usually lose weight easily, we're going to focus on all of the rest of us: the endomorphsof the world.

Endomorph Body Type

Endomorphs are usually described as curvaceous, full-figured, small-waisted and pear shaped.

They usually carry their weight in the thighs, hips andstomach rather than being evenly distributed throughout the body.

This kind of fat distribution can make it harder to lose weight than with the other body types.

Famous Endomorphs

If you're reading this because you identify as an endomorph, you're in good company!

Some of the world's most beautiful and celebrated women have been endomorphs.

Think Marilyn Monroe, Beyonce, Jennifer Lopez, Sophia Loren, Lana Turner, Elizabeth Taylor, Jayne Mansfield, Salma Hayek and Sophia Vergara, to name a few.

Is it Harder for an Endomorph to Lose Weight?

Endomorphs usually have a higher percentage of body fat along with less muscle mass, but that doesn't necessarily make them obese.

It does however, make endomorphs more sensitive to calorie consumption than the other body types.

According to somatotype research, endomorphs have slower metabolisms than ectomorphs and mesomorphs.

And that slower metabolism can cause extra calories to be converted to body fat.

If that isn't bad enough, endomorphs usually have a degree of carbohydrate sensitivity and may be more sensitive to insulin than the other body types.

Because of this insulin sensitivity, high carbohydrate foods are more quickly converted to sugar and are more likely to be stored as fat.

But don't despair – knowledge is power and you can fight back using a easy to follow endomorph diet plan.

Best Endomorph Diet Plan

Endomorphs have to watch what they eat more than the other body types.

Generally, a paleo-like diet, where each meal is built around protein, vegetables, and healthy fat is the best way for endomorphs to eat.

Because endomorphs can be carbohydrate and insulin sensitive, the best plan for this body type also focuses on lowering their intake of simple carbohydrates while upping their protein and healthy fat intake.

Best Macros for an Endomorph

Try to stick to a 30% Carbohydrate – 35 % Protein and 35% Fat balance with foods from the following categories:

Include Protein at EVERY Meal

As an endomorph, make sure you're eating lean protein with every meal you eat. Protein makes you feel full and takes longer to digest than other foods.

• Lean meat

• Fish

• Eggs

• Beans

• Nuts and seeds

• Protein powder

Carbs: Eat Lots of Vegetables

Focus on the "right" kind of carbs.

Most carbs should come from vegetables, the non-starchy, high-fiber kind. High fiber whole grains are also a good choice.

• Spinach

• Kale

• Broccoli

• Cauliflower

These carbohydrates are also considered the "right" kind for endomorphs.

• Fruits in moderation (fruits contain lots of sugar- try berries or green apples)

33

- Brown Rice

- Quinoa

- Oats

Eat A High-Quality Fat at Every Meal

Fat makes you feel full and good quality fats are healthy too!

Add healthy oil to your salad dressing, eat avocados in a delicious guacamole, saute veggies in grass-fed butter or coconut oil.

Foods to Avoid on the

Endomorph Diet

- Olive oil

- Avocados and avocado oil

- Grass-fed butter

- Coconut oil

- Nuts/seeds

- Cheese

Simple Carbohydrates to Avoid

- White bread

- White rice

- Pasta

• Cereal

Foods to Avoid if to Lose Weight as an Endomorph

• Fruit juice

• Cookies, crackers, and snack foods

• Soda

• Processed foods and added sugars

How an Endomorph Should Exercise

Endomorphs usually have a difficult time losing fat with diet alone.

So along with the endomorph diet plan, a regular combination of cardio and weight training is essential to boost your metabolism and keep the extra body fat at bay.

Muscle building can come easily for this body type, but endomorphs have to work harder to stay lean.

Cardio for Endomorphs

If you're an endomorph, you should concentrate on combining bursts of fat burning exercise, like HIIT (high intensity interval training), with longer steady-state cardio sessions.

Aim for 2 to 3 HIIT sessions per week for no more than 30 minutes per workout.

As for cardio, try to incorporate 30-60 minutes of cardio two to three days a week.

Weight Training for Endomorphs

Weight training can help build and maintain muscle which boosts your metabolism even after your workouts.

The more muscle your body has, the the more fat it can burn for fuel.

Focus on large muscle groups, compound exercises which use multiple muscle groups at one time, and circuit training with only short amounts of rest time between sets.

Stay Moving

For an endomorph workout at home, try to stay active even when you're not working out!

Anytime you can add activity to your day, you'll be helping your metabolism burn that fat.

Walk your dog, bike with your kids to the park, stretch while you're watching TV – any physical activity is beneficial!

One Last Tip to Boost the Endomorph Diet Plan

Eat slowly at meals! If you're an endomorph you may be carb sensitive so chew your food thoroughly and let your saliva do its job.

A study of Swedish families indicated that the biggest factor determining variations in BMI between family members had to do with a particular enzyme found in saliva.

Sounds confusing, but all it really means is that the longer you chew your food, the longer this important enzyme has to start breaking down the starch in your foods.

Conclusion

Understanding your body type, especially if you are an endomorph, and following the guidelines of the endomorph diet plan can help you meet your fitness goals while you get rid of those extra pounds.

Eat according to the recommendations above, chew your food well and keep moving!

Try Intermittent Fasting if You're an Endomorph

Intermittent fasting is one of the best ways I've found to lose weight. If you're curious, download my free guide for beginners and see if intermittent fasting can work for you too!

The Endomorph Diet Plan

As with any body type, I will tell you that roughly 80% of your results are coming how, what, and when you eat and the rest is from exercise.

In other words, you cannot out train a shitty diet so don't even try.

For the endomorph, diet is even more critical because you can't eat like the other body types and see positive results. The problem is that your body has a tendency to store fat at a much higher rate than the others.

The typical American diet is absolutely atrocious for the endomorph. Filled with processed foods, sugars, enriched products, chemicals, and hormone and anti-biotic laced products, it's a struggle to avoid these foods because they are so readily available and we so accustomed to eating them.

Know Your Macros

One key to success is going to be understanding your macronutrients (macros) and knowing how to balance them. This is extremely important for the endomorph.

Again, the normal diet we are eating is terrible for the endo and we can see by the macro breakdown that most of our calories are coming from carbohydrates. This spells disaster for the endomorph.

One of the best things you can do for yourself is to start tracking all your food. Do it for a week to start and I guarantee you'll be amazed at what you see.

In my experience, most people greatly over or underestimate their caloric intake and therefore, have no idea what their BMR is. How can you expect to drop body fat when you don't have any idea how many calories you need? You can't. It ends up being a guessing game and most of you are guessing wrong.

But don't beat yourself up, this is an easy fix. Start by downloading an app called MyFitnessPal and start tracking today. I'm serious, it's that important!

To find your BMR, use a tool called the Harris-Benedict Formula. Input your age, weight, and height and you will get a number. You will then multiply this number (your BMR) by your activity level to determine how many calories your body requires to maintain your current weight. You can then either reduce that number by 10-20% for fat loss or increase it by 10-20% for weight gain.

As far as your specific macros, there is no one answer as everyone has different levels of sensitivities, but a good starting point would be something like:

- 30-35% carbs

- 30-35% protein

- 30-35% fat

This low carb number will be a challenge for many endomorphs since they are typically used to eating a very high carb diet. You can expect to have an energy crash for a week or two, but after that, you'll feel 10X better.

Your main focus is to keep protein levels high. If nothing else, get your protein in every day.

Nutritional Rules to Live by

• Limit sugars, breads, pastas, cereals, crackers, and other heavy starches. Also remove white flour and byproducts.

• Eat a shitload of fibrous vegetables.

• Limit alcohol. They are empty calories and your body doesn't need them.

• Aim to eat a lean protein at every meal, preferably 25-35 grams. Not only is protein the most satiating macronutrient, it is critical for building the muscle you desperately need.

• Eat fat. Many endomorphs make the mistake of severely limiting or trying to eliminate fat because they think it will make them fatter. Not the case at all. In fact, healthy fats like nuts and nut butter, oils, fish oils, avocados, are crucial to the fat burning process.

• Take fish oil supplements if you don't eat enough fish. Fish oil has been shown to have a positive effect of many deadly diseases like coronary disease, Type 2 Diabetes, and high blood pressure, that are common among overweight and obese people, and as you know, many endomorphs fall into this category.

Insulin Issues

Insulin, which is a hormone that controls how your body absorbs sugar (and ultimately uses it for energy production), becomes an issue when you have an intolerance or sensitivity to carbohydrates.

As an endo, your body just isn't as good at using insulin to reduce the sugar in your bloodstream, which is one reason why eating sugary foods and high glycemic Index (GI) starchy carbs is a bad idea.

Eating high fiber, low GI foods may be a good idea and can help to keep blood sugars stable. These include:

• Whole grains like brown rice or quinoa.

• Starches like oatmeal or sweet potatoes.

• Fruits. Raspberries, strawberries, mangoes, apples, and bananas are best.

• Vegetables, especially green vegetables. Spinach, artichokes, kale, broccoli, and beets are excellent choices.

Many endomorphs also tend to have a slight to moderate carbohydrate intolerance. What this means is that your body will react poorly to excess carb intake and likely store it as fat versus burning it for energy.

This means that keeping your cab intake low (30-35% of total calories) is probably a good approach.

One caveat to the carb rule is that the endomorph should always eat carbs after a workout.

The Paleo Diet

As I've mentioned before, I am not a big believer in severely reducing or eliminating entire food groups, but there is something to be said for the success of the Paleo Diet.

First off, I've gone Paleo and it worked amazingly well. I have had clients eat Paleo style with great results as well. I'm not going to get into all the specifics and if you read this post, you'll learn everything you need to know about it.

Why I think it's a good idea to at least try it for 6 weeks or so is because it eliminates all the shit from your diet and as an endomorph, you NEED to remove it!

Basically your diet revolves around the following:

• Lean meats

• Fish and other seafood

• Eggs

• Fresh fruits and vegetables

• Healthy fats like nuts, seeds, and oils

These are all healthy things and while I'm not recommending you do or do not go on the Paleo, it's definitely with looking into it further, especially if you are struggling with carb intake.

Other Diets

I hate diets. I hate that they represent a short-term solution to a long-term need. Diets are temporary and more often than not, cause more harm than good when it comes to healthy fat loss.

Consider this example:

Smith is a 40 year old guy and an endomorph. He knows he needs to lose 30 pounds and is desperate to try something that works. He hears from his friend that a diet he recently tried helped him lose 35 pounds so Smith decides to give it a shot.

Here's what happens:

• Smith starts his diet at 200 pounds and has 18% body fat (this translates to 164 pounds of lean body mass (LBM) and 36 pounds of fat).

• He starts eating 1,500 calories per day based on the diet guidelines, although he is used to eating much more than that.

- In 8 weeks, he loses 21 pounds and is ecstatic! His body fat has also dropped to 15%.

- He feels like he's succeeded at his goal, but when we look at the numbers, we see something entirely different.

- Bob now weighs 179 pounds and has 15% body fat. This translates to 152 pounds of LBM and 27 pounds of fat. He has lost 9 pounds of fat, which is great, but he has also lost 12 pounds of muscle, which is terrible.

- Now Smith starts eating his normal 2,000 calories per day and within 12 weeks, has gained all his weight back.

- He is now 200 pounds at 20% body fat and has 159 pounds of LBM and 41 pounds of fat.

- He is now worse off than when he started, has a slower metabolism, and will find it harder to lose weight in the future

As you can see, this can wreak havoc on your body and when you "diet" frequently (AKA yo-yo dieting), it can be catastrophic for your body.

This scenario is extremely common and is caused by the diet industry's desire to make money. They don't give a shit about our health; they want to sell books, programs, and products.

The reason this model sells is because it produces results. Anyone can and will lose weight when given a low calorie diet, which most diets are in some capacity.

Quick results sell. Long and challenging doesn't.

But you shouldn't care about quick results. You should focus on making a permanent change to how you eat, move, and live.

The Endomorph Training Plana

Now that you know how important diet is for you, it's time to discuss the second piece of the puzzle; training.

As an endo, your body does not want to be lean and muscular. It wants to stay comfortable and be round and soft. Getting it to do what you want will require dedication, consistency, and a shit ton of hard work.

But if you do it, you can virtually "reset" your body type to be geared more towards a different one.

Rule one for any endomorph is to move more. Inactivity is your nemesis and living a sedentary life is the devil. Strength training is your savior and without it, you may live the rest of your life looking like one of the Teletubbies.

Your goal should be to reduce body fat, not weight. And the absolute best way to shed fat is to build lean muscle. This of course, is done through progressive strength training.

Our 90-Day Transformation Program, The Fit Dad Blueprint, includes 4 separate strength training programs so you can get started immediately if you're a newbie to fitness or if you've been training for years.

Strength Training

This is going to be the main staple for your exercise program. Everything starts here.

Since your primary goal is to build lean muscle tissue in order to drop body fat, increase your metabolism, and improve your overall health, you must strength train.

This means pushing your muscles way out of their comfort zones and overloading them to force growth. This can be done with weights or bodyweight exercises.

It's important to understand that all exercises are not created equal and using compound movements versus isolation ones can have a significant impact on your results and gains.

For the endomorph, the best use of your time and energy is using heavy, multi-joint compound exercise as the base for your strength workouts. Exercises like:

- Squats (front and back)

- Deadlifts

- Step ups

- Lunges

- Chest presses

- Overhead presses

- Pull ups and chin ups

- Rows

- Dips

Sample Workout

Here is an example of a proper strength training workout for an beginner to intermediate endomorph man:

• 3-4 days per week

• 2 upper body and 2 lower body workouts

• Reps are in the 8-12 range, meaning you cannot do 13. If you can, add weight

• Sets are 8-12 per body part

• Rest periods are 60 seconds

Upper body workout:

• Dumbbell chest press: 3 X 10

- Dips: 3 X 8-10

- (Incline) Pushups: 3 X 12-15

- Assisted pullups: 4 X 8

- One arm dumbbell row: 4 X 8-10

- Barbell overhead shoulder press: 3 X 10-12

- Dumbbell shrugs: 3 X 10

- Kettlebell farmers carry: 2 X distance

Lower body workout

- Kettlebell front squats: 4 X 8-10

- Leg press: 3 X 10-12

- Dumbbell step ups: 3 X 10-12

- Dumbbell stiff leg deadlift: 3 X 10-12

- Weighted glute/hamstring bridge: 3 X 10-12

As you can see, these are all compound exercises, using multiple joints and muscles at once. Also note that I didn't include specific ab work because many of these exercises force the core to stabilize and work to maintain posture and stability.

This is also not a plan designed for anyone specific. I believe in individualization of all exercise programs and recommend you find a good trainer or coach to help set one up for your specific goals, abilities, and limitations.

HIIT

I love high intensity interval training. Call it circuit training, interval training, or metabolic conditioning, it's all pretty much lumped together. The goal being to use short, very intense bursts of energy followed by short rest periods.

The goal is to use this type of training to elicit a higher calorie burn, increase heart capacity, improve muscular endurance and strength, and reap the rewards of EPOC.

But this is hardcore shit and if you are deconditioned, this type of training is going to be extremely taxing. They key is to push yourself to your limits, not those of someone else. Your perceived rate of exertion will differ greatly from mine for example and you should always train for your goals.

Sample HIIT Workout

I'm a big fan of timed circuit training and use it often with my clients and for myself. Below is a sample workout that would be ideal for an endomorph who is at the beginner to intermediate stages of fitness proficiency.

• 25 minutes or less total

• The goal is to get your heart rate up to 85% of your max for short periods. You max HR can be found by the following equation: 220-your age=max heart rate.

• 2-3 timed rounds

• 20 to 30 seconds of work followed by 30-40 seconds of rest

• 60-90 second rest periods between rounds

Sample Workout

• Pushups

• Air squats (or jump squats)

• Burpees

• Medicine ball toss

• Dumbbell curl to shoulder press

- Alternating lunge with rotations

- Plank jacks

The key is intensity here. Push yourself as hard as you are capable of but make sure to read your body. This type of training can place a lot of stress on your central nervous system and can even make you feel nauseous or sick.

Remember to push yourself to your limits and your limits only. Don't worry about how fast or how many reps someone else is doing or what you think you should be doing.

Cardio

Normally I am not a fan of steady state cardio like running, jogging, cycling and prefer high intensity work. However, since your goal is to move as much as possible, I do recommend doing traditional cardio several times per week. Walking, in particular, is a fantastic activity for the endomorph.

Just keep in mind that just because you get to walk on a treadmill for an hour, doesn't mean you get to take it easy. Push yourself on that thing too! Use inclines, speed variations, and hell even walking backwards works!

Golden Rules of Fitness for an Endomorph.

Ten Things you must Do

1. Move more, sit less. That means a walk instead of watching Game of Thrones, sorry.

2. Strength train 2-4 times per week depending on your fitness level. You NEED to build muscle in order to lose body fat.

3. Use interval/HIIT type training to supplement your strength training. The benefits are numerous and include a faster metabolism and a longer window of burning more calories (EPOC).

4. Track your calories (at least for a while).

5. Give yourself a cheat meal every 3-4 days. This will help you from feeling trapped in a diet and give you a mental reprieve.

6. Reduce stress. Cortisol can fuck with your hormones and slow progress.

7. Drink 80-128 ounces of water each day.

8. Be consistent and track your progress. Know your body fat and retake your measurements every 6-8 weeks to ensure its moving in the right direction....down.

9. Eat small, frequent meals consisting of lean protein, fibrous carbs, and healthy fats.

10. Get support. Use a friend, gym buddy, or trainer to help with motivation and to keep you on point.

Follow these 10 things and you will make progress, this I know. You don't have to do all of them right now, but you do need to do some of them.

Now get to work!

You Can Do This!

Focusing on just diet or just exercise is always a bad idea, but even more so for the endomorph. You must use both for things together for change to happen.

If you follow this guide, you will see results but be patient because it may take time. You didn't get soft and doughy overnight so you can't reasonably expect to reverse it overnight.

Remember, it's not about losing a bunch of weight, it's about adopting a healthy lifestyle that you can sustain.

This is the exact method I teach in our 90-Day Transformation Program, The Fit Dad Blueprint, and you'll get a step-by-step exercise and nutrition plan to help you shed some of that body and belly fat.

There is no reason to spend the rest of your life feeling fat, cursed by the metabolism Gods, or resigned to being called "big boned". You can make huge changes starting right now and some day you may look in the mirror and see a lean, muscular mesomorph staring back at you.

Printed in Great Britain
by Amazon